Plant Based Diet Cookbook

Healthy, Simple Whole Food Recipes to Reactivate Your Body and Awaken Your Taste Buds

Amellia Fox

Table of Contents

Introduction

You may be reading this book because you've tried countless fad diets that have failed miserably, tasted terrible, or were unachievable with their strict set of daily rules. Or, you may just be interested in a healthy lifestyle switch, one that benefits yourself and the environment. Either way, you're sure to gain some vital pieces of information and delectable recipe ideas from this book.

The following chapters will touch on the basics of a plant-based diet in a simple, easy-to-read format. As you discover this diet, you will quickly begin to see that this is more than just a simple change of food intake, but a positive and sustainable lifestyle change. You will also discover an array of simple yet broadly colorful recipes that will help you physically pave the way to your best self.

The plant-based diet is one of those lifestyle changes that once you gain momentum, it is quite easy to keep going, versus other diets that become complicated when trying to navigate past the beginning phases and permanently incorporate into your daily consumptions.

If you are ready to make a significant change in the way you fuel your body, then please do not hesitate trying some of these recipes. Even if you just start with a smoothie a few times a week or a simple clean eating bowl, you will feel a significant difference in your energy levels and mood almost immediately. This diet is utilized by many different individuals around the world, and is fast becoming the most popular way of eating to secure a healthy body and mind.

It's time to reactivate your body and awaken your taste buds!

The Plant-Based Diet Explained

The Plant-Based Diet is a whole-food diet that is based around minimizing and/or avoiding the consumption of meat products and dairy products - essentially any animal products or animal byproducts, and also highly refined/processed foods. *It encourages the consumption of unrefined, whole plants and minimally refined plant-based foods.* In other words, it is all about devouring vegetables, fruits, nuts, seeds, whole grains, tubers, and legumes in their most natural state. As you have probably already guessed, the plant-based diet is a form of Veganism, however there are many variations of this way of eating, you can tailor the diet to suit your needs, likes and dislikes.

A plant-based diet centers around bringing back the good ole ways of eating. Humankind thrived for thousands of years on a plant-based diet, and despite what you may be thinking, it is a satisfying and tasty way of getting the vitamins and nutrients our bodies require. But rest assured, this does not mean that you will only be eating leafy greens and other veggies. While greens are an important component in a plant-based diet, they are not the only main source of energy. You may have heard several stories of failure from those who have tried out one of these diets, because they are under the assumption that leafy greens were the only main food source they should be consuming. This is not the case; a multitude of delicious food items make up the foundation of a plant-based diet not just your stock standard kale and broccoli!

You are most likely pretty used to a meat substance taking center stage on your dinner plate, which may be one of the biggest hurdles new plant-based 'dieters' face when first starting this way of eating. Instead, a good portion of your plate should contain starch-based foods, such as legumes, grains and tubers, which we call 'starchy plant-food sources'. You may have been taught starch-based foods are unhealthy, but in reality, that is far from the truth. What makes starch-based food items unhealthy are the methods in which we prepare them, typically using a lot of unhealthy oils and dairies, and also the types of starch-based foods we choose to eat.

The recipes shown in this book will be Vegan in nature, however as mentioned above feel free to tailor the recipes to your desire. If you wish to follow a plant-based diet as closely as possible, the first step is cutting out meat and substituting it with plant-based food items that will be shown in the recipes to follow. Once you have successfully eliminated poultry and red meats from your diet, you are considered a 'pescatarian', meaning you still consume seafood. Once you erase seafood from your diet, you are officially a vegetarian. If you still wish to consume dairy products and eggs, you are known as a "lacto-ovo vegetarian" - which does sound pretty fancy!

Once you have erased all animal protein from your diet, it's time to slowly start removing diary and eggs as well. Eliminating dairy from the diet is the hardest step for many individuals, since it is in SO many consumables. While there are great alternatives for your daily glass of milk, people love cheese and hate to rid themselves of it. Thankfully, there are many cheese substitutes to choose from as well. *A rule of thumb for a positive mindset: focus on all the amazing things you will be fueling your body with, not what you are giving up, but what you are gaining.*

We are going to delve into our amazing MVP's of a plant-based diet in the next chapter, which make-up a powerhouse diet. If you wish to read more about the basics of a plant-based diet and the compelling benefits please refer to my previous book ***Plant Based Diet for Beginners***.

The MVP's of a Plant-Based Diet

In order to be successful in the beginning stages of a plant-based diet, you must be aware of the array of items that *are* highly encouraged to consume, especially since we are cutting out or at least minimizing the intake of animal proteins, we need to make sure our bodies are provided with key nutrients. We are going to rehash some of the **Most Valuable Players** of a plant-based diet, across the categories of Legume and Vegetables, Nuts and Seeds and Fruits which we discussed in my previous book (along with some new additions), and also add in a few more categories – herbs, spices and oils!

Legumes and Vegetables

- **Lentils:** These guys can be pretty simply added to a variety of meals and are a loaded with essential protein and fiber, packed into a low-calorie package. In just a half a cup there are 9 whopping grams of protein! You can make them as a side dish or use them as a substitute for meat or create delicious dips! *Bonus: Great at lowering cholesterol and promoting heart health!*

- **Edamame**: These delicious cooked soybeans are amazing sources of protein, with 18 grams being packed in just one cup. You can eat them as an appetizer or add them into side dishes and stir-fry meals. Opt for purchasing ones with a certified organic seal, since many soybeans within the U.S. are modified genetically.

- **Lima Beans**: Lima beans offer a great side dish to a variety of main courses or can be added to a hefty salad or soup. They are packed with 7.3 grams of protein per serving! *Bonus: They contain an amino acid called leucine, which helps in muscle synthesis.*

- **Black Beans:** These beans are another great multi-use veggie. They are packed with Vitamin B6, potassium, folate, and fiber. Every serving has 7.6 grams of protein. They can easily be used to make yummy veggie burgers, vegan brownies or a killer vegan Mexican meal!

- **Chickpeas:** Chickpeas are highly versatile and can easily be utilized in a vast array of dishes. They are infamous for making delicious hummus! They are loaded with 6 grams of protein per serving, and they are easy. You can also use chickpea water as an egg replacement known as aquafaba!

- **Spinach:** Spinach is one of the most superb green veggies out there. Each serving is packed with 3 grams of protein and is a highly encouraged component of the plant-based diet.

- **Kale:** Kale is the latest superfood of the Vegan world. It is a favorite when deciding to eliminate meat from your diet as it is very high in iron, vitamin K and potassium. It is also extremely high in fibre and vitamin A.

- **Broccoli:** Once cooked, you receive 2 grams of

protein per serving of broccoli, along with a nice helping of fiber. It is also a good source of calcium and zinc.

- **Eggplant:** Eggplant has a variety of vital vitamins and minerals within it's compound. It is high in folic acid, vitamin C, manganese and vitamin K. It aids weight lose and cognitive function. Eggplant is a great meat replacement in a lasagna!

- **Zucchini:** This commonly known vegetable (which botanically is considered a fruit!), promotes healthy eyes and heart function. They are high in folate and potassium. They are great to use as a substitute for spaghetti/noddles, just grab a spiralizer and get spiralizing!

- **Brussels Sprouts:** 2 grams of protein per serving is not the only healthy component of this misunderstood vegetable. They also offer consumers a good dose of potassium and Vitamin K.

- **Cauliflower:** This vegetable is an extremely high source of vitamin A, vitamin B1, B2 and B3. It is so high in vitamin A that it alone makes up 85% of your recommended daily vitamin A intake. It has even been said that it can be used as a stress reliever!

- **Potatoes:** Potatoes are a great starchy source of potassium and protein. They are pretty inexpensive if you are one that is watching their budget. *Bonus: Very heart healthy!*

Fruits

- **Avocado:** Avocados are known as miracle fruits in

the world of Veganism. They are a true super-fruit and incredibly beneficial. They are one of the best things to eat if you are looking to incorporate more fatty acids in your diet. They are also loaded with 20 various minerals and vitamins. Plus, they are easy to incorporate into dishes all throughout the day!

- **Grapefruit:** Contrary to popular belief, oranges are not your best bet when attempting to add more Vitamin C into your diet. Pick up a grapefruit instead, for they have 50% more than the average orange! They are also loaded with potassium, fiber, and Vitamin A. *Bonus: Assists with arthritis. Double Bonus: Great remedy for oily skin!*

- **Pineapple:** This juicy and delicious fruit can be devoured in an array of ways, which means it is a good item to incorporate into meals. *Bonus: Since pineapples are full of anti-inflammatory nutrients, they aid in reducing stroke and heart attacks. Double Bonus: Pineapples have also been known to increase fertility!*

- **Blueberries:** These guys are a delectable treat that is easily incorporated into many dishes. They are packed with antioxidants and Vitamin C. *Bonus: Blueberries have been proven to promote eye health and slow macular degeneration.*

- **Pomegranate:** Pomegranates are one of those fruits that are multi-purpose, consumers can utilize both the seeds and the juice. They are filled with antioxidants and potassium. *Bonus: Promote heart and cardiovascular health and are known to lower* *cholesterol.*

- **Apples:** "An apple a day keeps the doctor away" is far from just an old wives' tale! Apples are loaded with antioxidants and are a delicious low-calorie snack. *Bonus: Protect the health of the brain and heart. Double Bonus: Assist in lowering cholesterol. Triple bonus: Aid in weight loss. Quadruple bonus: Aid in oral health. In other words, pick up an apple if you are in need of a snack.*

- **Kiwi:** This tart fruit is loaded with Vitamins E and C, along with many types of antioxidants. They are loaded with fiber and have a low-calorie count, which makes them a guilt-free snack. *Bonus: Promote eye health. Double Bonus: Lowers the chances of cancer. Triple Bonus: Aids in weight loss!*

- **Mango:** Mangos contain 50% of the daily Vitamin C you should consume and consist of beta-carotene, a nutrient that the body converts into Vitamin A which aid in bone and immune health.

- **Lemons:** Lemons are popularly known as harboring loads of Vitamin C, but are also excellent sources of folate, fiber, and antioxidants. *Bonus: Helps lower cholesterol. Double Bonus: Reduces risk of cancer and high blood pressure.*

- **Cranberries:** Cranberries are known for their levels of Vitamin C, but many do not know that they also a great source of fiber and contain more antioxidants than other fruits and veggies. *Bonus: They are a great boost to the immune system. Double Bonus: Promote urinary tract health. Triple*

Bonus: Assist the body in absorbing magnesium and Vitamins E and K.

Nuts and Seeds

- **Peanuts & Peanut Butter:** Peanuts are quite an agreeable super-food from the points of views of plant-based and meat-eaters alike. Both peanuts and peanut butter contain 7 grams of protein per serving and can be consumed in a variety of ways. While most types of peanut butter are vegan, make sure to read the label, for some contain honey..

- **Chia Seeds:** Chia seeds are widely known to the vegan world and can be sprinkled on just about anything and everything. They are an amazing source of calcium, fiber, protein, and Vitamin C. Add them to your smoothies, breakfast meals and clean eating bowls for an extra bang!

- **Pumpkin Seeds:** Pumpkin seeds are popularly known as a yummy snack, and can also be easily incorporated into soups, yogurt, salads, and more! They are loaded with iron, Vitamins C, E, and K, and essential omega-3s.

- **Almonds:** Almonds are commonly used as a substitute for dairy in the vegan world. They are packed with lots of good things, such as B vitamins, iron, potassium, phosphorus, magnesium, protein, and fiber! *Bonus: They are known to strengthen bones and lower cholesterol. Double Bonus: They are great for hair and skin!*

- **Flaxseeds:** These guys are awesome add-ins to

most plant-based meals since they can be ground up and added to things such as cookies, muffins, bread, cereal, oatmeal, and smoothies. They are packed with B vitamins, zinc, magnesium, and protein. *Bonus: They aid in digestion and assist with suppressing appetite, which aids in weight loss!*

- **Sesame Seeds:** Sesame seeds can be easily added to crackers, bread, salads, and stir-fry meals. *Bonus: Help in lowering cholesterol and high blood pressure. Double bonus: Help with asthma, arthritis, and migraines!*

- **Sunflower Seeds:** These seeds can be used to make butter, making a great alternative to dairy. They contain B vitamins, iron, Vitamin E, and lots of healthy fats.

- **Walnuts:** Walnuts have been proven to boost your metabolism, regulate sleep, assist in clear skin, heart function and bone health.

- **Cashews:** These nuts are low in sodium and are packed with flavor, which is why they are an infamous source of protein and vitamins in Veganism.

- **Brazil Nuts:** These nuts are high in B vitamin, iron, fiber, and protein.

- **Pine Nuts:** Pine nuts are low in calories and can be easily paired with many types of dishes. You can bake them into foods or create decadent sauces out of them. They are filled with potassium, magnesium, iron, and many antioxidants.

Oils

- **Coconut Oil:** Coconut oil is full of healthy fats that are absorbed easily in the human body. It is a go-to when it comes to Vegan cooking since it is a great substitute for butter and vegetable oils. It can also be used topically, in treating hair and skin. *Bonus: Contains fatty acids that aid in weight loss. Double Bonus: Strengthens the immune system.*

- **Olive Oil:** This oil is a main source of dietary fat in a variety of diets. It contains many vitamins and minerals that play a part in reducing the risk of stroke and lowers cholesterol and high blood pressure and can also aid in weight loss. It is best consumed cold, as when it is heated it can lose some of its nutritive properties (although it is still great to cook with – extra virgin is best), many recommend taking a shot of cold oil olive daily! *Bonus: if you don't like the taste or texture add a shot to your smoothie.*

- **Grape Seed Oil:** Formed from the seeds of grapes, its clean and light taste is what makes it a popular component in salad dressings, home-made mayonnaise, and baked goods. It contains high levels of omega-6 fatty acids. *Bonus: Great part of a skin and hair beauty regimen.*

- **Rice Bran Oil:** This oil is a popular choice in the Vegan world of cooking, especially when it comes to making stir-fry dishes. It is full of antioxidants and has a significant amount of Vitamin E. It can maintain its nutritive properties even at very high temperatures, which is amazing! *Bonus: Rice bran oil has been shown to lower cholesterol. Double Bonus: Has been proven to lower assist with the symptoms of menopause in women.*

- **Avocado Oil:** Avocados themselves are ranked within the top five of the healthiest foods on the planet, so you know that the oil that is produced from them is too. It is loaded with healthy fats and essential fatty acids. Like race bran oil it is perfect to cook with as well! *Bonus: Helps in the prevention of diabetes and lowers cholesterol levels.*

- **Flaxseed Oil:** This oil contains omega-3 fatty acids and can aid in weight loss, muscle pain relief, inflammation and prevent premature aging. This oil is not to be used when cooking, but can be added to cold beverages such as tea, juice and smoothies.

Herbs and Spices

- **Cinnamon:** This spice is an absolute powerhouse and is considered one of the healthiest, beneficial spices on the plant. It can be used in a variety of dishes, and is a fantastic addition to your daily smoothie. It's widely known for its medicinal properties. This spice is loaded with powerful antioxidants and is popular for its anti-inflammatory properties. It can reduce heart disease and lower blood sugar levels.

- **Ginger:** Ginger is famous for being not only delicious but extremely healthy as well. It is packed with bioactive compounds and nutrients that make it a great fuel for both your mind and body. It is also known to assist with nausea.

- **Turmeric:** Turmeric is one of the most nutritional supplements known to mankind. Yellow in color, it is known for treating anti-inflammatory ailments and is loaded with antioxidants that strengthen the brain.

- **Basil:** A popular choice of seasoning in many types of cooking, basil is best known for its part in Italian cuisine. It aids in anti-inflammatory ailments and is loaded with antibacterial properties, aiding in fending off sickness.

- **Sage:** Sage is a plant with a well-known aroma. It is packed with bacteria-killing capabilities and is used in many antiseptics. It is also loaded with a variety of oils that provide the body with nutrients that can easily be absorbed by the body when consumed.

- **Thyme:** Thyme is an evergreen shrub that has been utilized both in the culinary arts and medicinally for thousands of years. Its stems can be used fresh or dried and is a great add in to many dishes, especially sauces and soups. It's loaded with antioxidants and is known to build the immune system and improve circulation in the body.

- **Oregano:** Oregano is an herb that has a pleasant aroma, loaded with anti-bacterial properties and antioxidants. It is utilized in flavoring sauces and baked into many types of bread. It's proven to help treat diabetes, cancer, and osteoporosis.

- **Chives:** Chives are a very nutrient-dense food,

meaning they have a low-calorie count but are packed with antioxidants, vitamins, and minerals. Chives have been shown to improve mood.

Now that we've covered some excellent plant-based food items, that should be strongly considered when planning meals, we are ready to dive right in and get cooking. The next few chapters will cover smoothies, clean eating bowls, soup, stews and curries, breakfast, lunch and dinner meals, side dishes and snacks and desserts and treats! *Please note: serve quantities listed are based on an average person's consumption, they may vary from individual to individual.*

Smoothies

Smoothies are a fantastic way to get your daily dose of essential vitamins and nutrients in, especially if you're on the go! Smoothies are also a fabulous way to hide food items such as herbs, spices, oils, supplements and vegetables that your taste buds may not love but your body sure does. You can use smoothies as a meal replacement, many love to have a smoothie instead of a heavy breakfast. Invest in a decent blender, and get started.

All Star Smoothie

Serves: one

Ingredients:

- 1 C. organic almond milk

- 1 banana

- ½ C. frozen berries

- 1 tsp. chia seeds

- ½ C. spinach or kale

- 1 tsp. ground cinnamon

- 1 tsp. ground ginger

- 1 tbsp. extra virgin olive oil

- 1 tsp. ground turmeric

Method:

- Peel Banana and cut up into four pieces.

- Pour all smoothie components into a blender, generally starting with a liquid first.

- Blend on high speed till the mixture reaches your desired consistency. Enjoy!

The Green Machine

Serves: one

Ingredients:

- 1 tbsp. coconut oil

- 1 C. coconut water

- 1 C. organic almond milk

- 2 kiwi fruits

- ½ C. spinach or kale

- 1 C. celery

- 1 tbsp. Spirulina

Method:

- Chop up the two kiwi fruits, you can decide whether to keep the skin on or not (the skin is very nutritious).

- Chop up the celery.

- Pour all smoothie components into a blender.

- Blend on high till you achieve the consistency you desire. Devour!

Summertime Squeeze

Serves: one

Ingredients:

- 3 cubes ice

- 1 C. coconut water

- 2 tbsp. aloe vera juice

- 1 C. watermelon

- ½ C. frozen strawberries

- ½ C. frozen mango

Method:

- Cut up watermelon into cubes.

- Pour all smoothie components into a blender.

- Blend on high till smoothie mixture reaches the consistency you desire.

Quinoa Raspberry Coconut Smoothie

Serves: one

Ingredients:

- 1 C. organic almond milk

- 2 tbsp. shredded coconut

- 2 tbsp. dried goji berries

- ½ C. cooked quinoa

- 1 medjool date

- 1 C. raspberries

Method:

- Take out the pit from the date.

- Pour all smoothie components into a blender.

- Blend 30 seconds till mixture is smooth or reaches your desired consistency. Enjoy!

Spicy Banana Oat Smoothie

Serves: one

Ingredients:

- 1 C. organic almond milk

- ¼ tsp. ground turmeric

- ½ tsp. ground cinnamon

- ¼ tsp. ground ginger

- 1 banana

- ¼ C. rolled oats

Method:

- Peel and cut up banana in four pieces.

- Pour all smoothie components into a blender.

- Blend till mixture is smooth or reaches your desired consistency.

Green Apple Ginger Smoothie

Serves: one

Ingredients:

- 1 C. organic orange juice

- 2 tbsp. aloe vera juice

- 1 tbsp. chia or flax seeds

- ½ tsp. ground cinnamon

- 1 tsp. minced ginger root

- 1 banana

- 1 apple of choice

- 1 ½ C. kale

Method:

- Peel and cut up banana into four pieces.

- Cut and core apple.

- Pour smoothie components into the blender.

- Blend till smooth or till mixture reaches your desired consistency.

Blueberry Avocado Chia Smoothie

Serves: one

Ingredients:

- 1 C. organic almond milk
- ¼ tsp. vanilla powder
- 1 tbsp. chia seeds
- ½ ripe avocado
- 1 tsp. avocado oil
- 1 tsp. flaxseed oil
- 1 medjool date
- 1 C. blueberries

Method:

- Skin and pit avocado. Cut in half and place in a blender.

- Pour in remaining smoothie components into the blender.

- Blend 30 seconds till smooth or till mixture reaches desired consistency. Enjoy!

Very Berry Smoothie

Serves: one

Ingredients:

- 1 C. water
- 1 tsp. ground cinnamon
- Sprig of spearmint
- ½ C. pineapple
- ½ C. peaches
- ½ C. strawberries
- ½ C. blueberries
- 1 frozen banana
- ½ C. raspberries

Method:

- Pour all smoothie components into a blender with the exception of spearmint.
- Blend on high speed till the mixture turns out smooth.
- Serve in your favorite glass with a sprig of spearmint and a pinch of cinnamon. Enjoy!

Hidden Greens Chocolate Protein Smoothie

Serves: one

Ingredients:

- 1 ½ C. organic almond milk
- 1 tbsp. avocado
- 1 tsp. ground cinnamon
- 1 banana, frozen
- 2 tbsp. unsweetened cocoa powder
- 2 tbsp. hulled hemp seeds
- 2-3 dates
- 1 C. frozen kale
- Handful of ice

Method:

- Cut up banana into four pieces.
- Take out the pits from the dates.
- Pour all smoothie components into a blender.
- Blend on high till mixture is smooth.
- Adjust sweetness to your liking. Enjoy!

Butternut Cinnamon Date Smoothie

Serves: two

Ingredients:

- 1 C. + ½ C. organic almond milk
- 5-6 ice cubes
- 1 tsp. of ground cloves
- ½ tsp. ground ginger
- 1 ½ tsp. vanilla extract
- 1-2 tsp. ground cinnamon
- 1 tbsp. chia seeds
- 3-4 dates
- ¾ - 1 C. canned pureed squash

Method:

- Take out the pits from the dates.
- Add all smoothie components to a blender.
- Blend on high for 30 seconds or till mixture reaches desired consistency.
- Pour into two glasses and share with a friend or loved one!

Breakfast

Ricotta Pancakes with Peaches and Blueberries

Serves: two-four (depending on the size of your pancakes)

Ingredients:

- 4 peaches
- Punnet of blueberries
- 2 tbsp. coconut oil
- 1 tbsp. lemon juice
- 1 tsp. vanilla extract
- 1 C. organic almond milk
- ½ C. vegan & fat-free ricotta
- 1 tbsp. baking powder
- 1/4 tsp. stevia or 2 tbsp. brown sugar
- 1 ½ C. whole-grain flour

Method:

- Sift dry components together in a bowl.
- Whisk wet components together in a bowl.

- Mix dry and wet mixtures together in a larger bowl.

- Warm coconut oil in a skillet.

- Cook ¼ cup of pancake batter at a time.

- Top each pancake with peaches and blueberries and allow to simmer.

- Continue process until batter is gone.

- Serve with your favorite syrup and/or toppings if you wish.

Sweet and Salty Muesli Bark with Coconut Yogurt and Berries

Serves: one-two

Ingredients:

- 1 ½ C. whole-grain muesli

- ¼ C. shredded coconut

- ¼ C. dark non-dairy chocolate chips

- 1 C. frozen mixed berries

- 2 tbsp. agave nectar

- 2 C. coconut yogurt

- 1 tbsp. chia seeds

Method:

- Mix yogurt and agave together. Then add in berries, chocolate chips, and coconut. Combine well.

- With foil, line a tray. Pour mixture into the tray.

- Freeze at least 2 hours till frozen.

- Once frozen, use a knife to break apart bark. Enjoy!

Orange French Toast

Serves: four

Ingredients:

French Toast:

- 8 whole-grain bread slices

- ½ tbsp. orange zest

- 2 pinches of salt

- 1 tsp. cinnamon

- 2 tbsp. organic maple syrup

- 1 C. aquafaba (aka chickpea water - egg replacement)

- ½ C. ground almond flour

- 1 ½ C. organic almond milk

- ¼ C. sesame seeds

Berry Compote:

- 1 tsp. organic maple syrup

- 2 pureed cored apples (acting applesauce)

- 4 ½ ounces frozen blueberries and raspberries

Method:

- Ensure oven is preheated to 400 degrees. Put a wire rack on a baking tray.

- Mix salt, cinnamon, maple syrup, aquafaba, flour, and almond milk together. Pour into a shallow dish and stir in orange zest and sesame seeds.

- Warm up a skillet. Dip each slice of bread into cinnamon mixture and allow to soak for a few moments. Turn over each piece and repeat.

- Put in skillet and cook 2-3 minutes per side.

- Place toast on the rack and bake 10-15 minutes till crispy.

- Put cored apples into a food processor and blend.

- Mix maple syrup, applesauce, and berries in a blender. Blend till chunky.

- Serve toast topped with berry compote.

Chocolate Chip Coconut Pancakes

Serves: two-four (depending on the size of your pancakes)

Ingredients:

- 1/3 C. dark non-dairy chocolate chips

- 1 tsp. vanilla extract

- ¼ C. organic maple syrup

- 2 pureed cored apples (acting applesauce)

- 1 C. organic almond milk

- Pinch of salt

- 1 tbsp. baking powder

- 2 tbsp. unsweetened coconut flakes

- ¼ C. old-fashioned rolled oats

- 1 ¼ C. organic buckwheat flour

- 1 tbsp. flaxseeds

Optional:

- 1 banana

Method:

- Pour flaxseeds in a pan with ½ cup of water. Cook 3-4 till mixture appears stringy and sticky. Strain and set to side. Throw out seeds.

- Put cored apples into a food processor and blend.

- Mix together salt, baking powder, coconut flakes, oats, applesauce, and buckwheat flour.

- In another bowl, mix vanilla, syrup, applesauce, and almond milk together along with 2 tbsp of flaxseed water.

- Mix together dry and wet mixtures. Fold in chocolate chips.

- Pour 1/3 of a cup of pancake batter into a warmed up griddle. Cook 6-8 minutes on the first side, flip, and cook opposing side 5 minutes.

- Serve pancakes with sliced bananas if desired.

Chickpea Omelet with Pomegranates

Serves: two

Ingredients:

- 3 chopped green onions
- ½ tsp. baking soda
- 1/3 C. nutritional yeast
- ¼ tsp. pepper
- ¼ tsp. white pepper
- ½ tsp. garlic powder
- ½ tsp. onion powder
- 1 C. organic chickpea flour
- ¼ cup almonds
- 1 tbsp chia seeds
- 1 C. pomegranates

Ingredients:

- Mix baking soda, yeast, black and white pepper,

39

garlic powder, onion powder, and chickpea flour together. Then pour in 1 cup water and stir until smooth batter forms.

- Warm up a frying pan and pour batter into it as if you were making pancakes. Sprinkle a couple tbsp of green onions into the batter. Flip omelet. Let cook till brown, and flip again, cooking opposing side for 60 seconds.

- Serve omelets with almonds, chia seeds and pomegranates on top.

Apple Lemon Breakfast

Serves: two

Ingredients:

- ¼ tsp. cinnamon

- 2 tbsp. walnuts

- 1 tbsp. pumpkin seeds

- Juice of a lemon

- 5-6 pitted dates

- 4-5 apples of choice

Method:

- Core apples and slice into pieces.
- Pour half of lemon juice, ¾ of apples, cinnamon, walnuts, pumpkin seeds and dates into a food processor. Process till ground.

- Pour in remaining lemon juice and apples, pulsing till apples are shredded, and date mixture is distributed.

Cauliflower Breakfast Scramble

Serves: two

Ingredients:

- ¼ C. nutritional yeast
- 1-2 tbsp. soy sauce
- 3 minced garlic cloves
- ¼ tsp. cayenne pepper
- 1 ½ tsp. turmeric
- Pinch of salt
- 1 head of cauliflower
- 2 C. sliced mushrooms
- 1 green bell pepper
- 1 red bell pepper
- 1 red onion

Method:

- Cut up onion, bell peppers, and cauliflower. Sauté in a skillet for 7-8 minutes till onions become translucent. Pour in 1-2 tbsp. water in to avoid veggies sticking to the pan.

- Place cauliflower florets into the pan and cook 5-6 minutes till tender.

- Add yeast, soy sauce, garlic, cayenne, turmeric, pepper, and salt. Cook 5 minutes until fragrant.

Whole Grain Blueberry Muffins

Serves: two

Ingredients:

- 1 C. blueberries

- 1 ½ tsp. vanilla extract

- ½ C. organic maple syrup

- 2 pureed cored apples (acting applesauce)

- ¼ tsp. baking soda

- 2 C. whole-grain flour

- 1 tsp. organic apple cider vinegar (with the 'mother')

- 1 tbsp. flaxseeds

- 2/3 C. organic almond milk

Method:

- Ensure oven is preheated to 350 degrees. Use cupcake liners to prepare a muffin tin.

- Pour vinegar, flaxseeds, and almond milk into measuring cup and whisk quickly with a fork until foamy. Set to side.

- Put cored apples into a food processor and blend.

- Sift salt, baking soda, along with the flour. Within the center of dry mixture, create a well, and pour in milk mixture. Then add vanilla, syrup, and applesauce, combining well. Fold in berries.

- Fill each muffin liner ¾ of the way full.

- Bake 22-26 minutes.

Apple Walnut Breakfast Bread

Serves: four

Ingredients:

- ½ C. walnuts

- 1 tsp. cinnamon

- Pinch of salt

- ½ tsp. baking powder

- 1 tsp. baking soda

- 2 C. whole-grain flour

- 1 tbsp. ground flaxseeds

- 1/3 C. organic almond milk

- 1 tsp. stevia or ¾ C. brown sugar

- 2 pureed cored apples (acting applesauce)

Method:

- Ensure oven is preheated to 375 degrees.

- Put cored apples into a food processor and blend.

- Combine flaxseeds, almond milk, stevia/brown sugar, and applesauce together till smooth. Set to the side.

- Mix baking soda and powder, cinnamon along with salt.

- Combine dry and wet mixtures together. Stir in walnuts.

- Pour into a loaf pan.

- Bake 25-30 minutes till golden in color. Sit on a wire rack to cool before attempting to cut. Enjoy!

Brown Rice Breakfast Pudding

Serves: two

Ingredients:

- ¼ C. slivered almonds

- Pinch of salt

- ¼ C. raisins

- 1 tart apple

- 1 C. dates

- 1 tsp. chopped cloves

- 1 tsp. chopped chives

- 1 cinnamon stick

- 2 C. organic almond milk

- 3 C. brown rice

Method:

- Cook brown rice for 15-20 minutes in boiling water.

- Take pips out of dates.

- Mix dates, cloves, chives, cinnamon stick, almond milk, and rice together in a saucepan. Stir over low heat 12 minutes till it thickens.

- Take out cinnamon stick. Pour in salt, raisins, and apple. Mix well.

- Serve topped with toasted almonds.

Lunch

Lentil Tacos

Serves: two

Ingredients:

- 2 ½ C. organic vegetable broth
- 1 tsp. oregano
- 2 tsp. cumin
- 1 tbsp. chili powder
- ½ C. black beans
- 1 C. dried lentils
- 1 minced clove garlic
- 1 chopped onion
- 2 tsp. avocado oil
- ¼ C. salsa
- 2 whole-grain soft taco wraps
- *Optional salad items:*
- 1 chopped tomato
- ½ C. spinach

- 1 smashed avocado

- ¼ C. jalapenos (if you like that kick!)

Method:

- Warm up 1 tsp. avocado oil. Sauté onion and garlic together till tender.

- Pour in seasonings and rinsed lentils. Cook for 60 seconds, stirring well.

- Pour broth in and warm mixture till it boils.

- Turn down warm and put on the lid. Simmer 25-30 minutes till lentils are tender.

- Mash lentils a bit and stir in salsa.

- Rinse black beans and heat up in a frying pan with 1 tsp. avocado oil for 60 seconds.

- Serve in whole grain soft taco wraps with your favorite salad items or used the optional items mentioned above. Enjoy!

Cauliflower and Sweet Potato Bake

Serves: four

Ingredients:

- 1 tbsp. chopped parsley

- 1 slice of whole-grain sourdough bread

- ½ C. vegan grated cheese

- ½ C. sesame seeds

- 2 C. organic almond milk

- 3 tbsp. whole-grain flour

- 3 tbsp. coconut oil

- 2 tbsp. water

- 2 crushed cloves garlic

- 1 sliced leek

- 1 tsp. extra virgin olive oil

- 3 C. cauliflower florets

- 5 C. sweet potato

Method:

- Place sweet potato over hot water in a pan within a steamer basket. Cover and let simmer 8-10 minutes till tender. Put on a plate and set aside.

- Place cauliflower into the same steamer basket. Let steam 6-8 minutes until tender.

- Warm up extra virgin olive oil and place leek and garlic into the pan. Cook 2 minutes, stirring constantly. Pour water in, allow to cook 8 minutes till leek is tenderized.

- In an ovenproof dish, layer cauliflower, leek, and sweet potato.

- Melt coconut oil. Take pan off heat and mix in flour

- Put back on heat and stir 1 minute as you gradually add in almond milk. Allow to cook 6-7 minutes till the sauce becomes thick and begins to simmer.

- Pour sauce over veggies.

- Sprinkle vegan cheese and sesame seeds over it.

- Bake 25-30 minutes until golden brown. Sprinkle with parsley and enjoy!

Chickpea Quinoa Burgers

Serves: Two

Ingredients:

- ½ tsp. cayenne

- ½ tsp. cumin

- 1 tsp. curry

- ¼ C. organic chickpea flour

- 1 C. organic mixed frozen veggies

- Pinch of pepper and salt

- 2 tbsp. rice bran oil

- 1 C. cooked chickpeas

- 1 C. cooked quinoa

- Four whole-grain buns

Optional salad items:

- 1 chopped tomato

- Cut up pineapple

- Grated/shaved raw beetroot

- ½ C. spinach

- ¼ chopped onion

Method:

- Heat up the mixed frozen veggies in a frying pan with 1 tbsp. rice bran oil.

- Mix together all ingredients in a bowl till a thick burger mixture forms. With hands, form 6-8 burgers.

- Add 1 tbsp. rice bran oil into a warmed skillet. Cook burgers on each side till browned.

- Serve on top of the toasted whole-grain bun with your choice of salad items or incorporate the optional delicious toppings mentioned above.

Crispy Tofu and Rainbow Veggie Sushi

Serves: four

Ingredients:

- 2-3 tbsp. sesame seeds

- 1 tbsp. nutritional yeast

- 2 tbsp. low-sodium soy sauce

- 1 pack of organic tofu

- 1 red bell pepper

- 1 carrot

- 1 sliced avocado

- 1 pack toasted nori seaweed sheets

- 1/3 C. rice vinegar

- 3 tbsp. agave

- Pinch of salt

- 3 ½ C. water

- 2 C. brown sushi rice

Method:

- Ensure oven is preheated to 425 degrees. With parchment paper, line a baking sheet.

- Arrange tofu on the sheet. Drizzle tofu with soy sauce and sprinkle with yeast. Rub slices to ensure even coating.

- Bake 10 minutes per side, flipping once during the baking process. When they are golden, take out of the oven. Let cool. Cut into ½" wide strips.

- While tofu bakes, bring a pot of water and rice to boiling. Reduce heat and cover pot. Cook 10-15 minutes till moisture is absorbed. Allow to cool.

- Slice your veggies.

- Pour cold water into a bowl. Once rice is a bit cooled off, mix in agave, salt, and rice vinegar.

- Layout 1 piece of seaweed. Put 1 cup of rice on top. Put fingers in cold water and press rice to seaweed, making sure to spread to the edges.

- Lay out a small portion of veggies in the middle of the rice.

- Roll seaweed, tightly squeezing till you get to the end. Dip fingers in the water again and put on seaweed to seal the roll.

- Repeat process till you use all ingredients. To serve, sprinkle with toasted sesame seeds. Enjoy!

Coconut Butter Veggie Rice Noodles

Serves: four

Ingredients:

- ¼ C. chopped cilantro

- Pinch of salt and pepper

- ½ tsp. turmeric

- 1 tbsp. rice vinegar

- 1 tbsp. agave

- 1 tbsp. soy sauce

- 2 tbsp. almond butter

- 1 can organic coconut milk

- 2 C. chopped spinach
- 2 C. broccoli florets
- 1 sliced carrot
- 3-4 sliced mushrooms
- 1" peeled/chopped ginger
- 1 tsp. coconut oil
- 2 chopped cloves garlic
- 1 sliced shallot
- 8 ounces organic rice noodles

Method:

- Prepare rice noodles. Drain and rinse. Set aside.
- Sauté ginger, garlic, and onion in a frying pan with 1 tsp. coconut oil 1-2 minutes.
- Pour in veggies and combine. Cook 1-2 minutes.
- Pour in coconut milk. Cook 2-3 minutes till veggies soften.
- Combine nut butter with a bit of warmed water till creamy.
- Add in pepper, salt, turmeric, agave, vinegar, soy sauce, and almond butter mixture. Combine well.
- Toss veggies and sauce well with tongs.
- Add herbs.

Mega Lentil Burger

Serves: two

Ingredients:

- ¾ - 1 C. coarse cornmeal
- ¼ tsp. cayenne
- 1 tsp. salt
- 3 tbsp. flaxseeds
- 1 tbsp. mustard
- 1/3 C. tomato paste
- ½ C. chopped walnuts
- 1 C. chopped sweet potato
- 1 clove of garlic
- 1 ¾ C. dried lentils
- 1 C. brown rice
- ¼ lettuce

Method:

- Cook lentils and rice separately in boiling water on a stovetop until ready.

- Ensure oven is preheated to 450 degrees. With parchment paper, line a tray and lightly grease with olive oil.

- Combine walnuts, sweet potato, garlic, and onion in a food processor till mixture is consistently uniform. Add in lentils and rice and process. Pour into a mixing bowl.

- Add pepper, salt, cayenne, flax meal, mustard, and tomato paste. Mix well.

- Pour cornmeal in, mixing till the mixture becomes thick.

- Form patties with your hand.

- Place patties on the tray. Bake 15-20 minutes till slightly crisp.

- Break of decent sized lettuce leaves to use as a the wrap and top with your favorite sauce if you wish.

Orzo Salad with Herbs

Serves: two

Ingredients:

- ½ - ¾ C. organic red wine vinaigrette

- ¼ C. chopped basil

- ¼ C. chopped chives

- ¾ C. chopped onion

- 1 ½ C. cherry tomatoes

- 1 C. rinsed garbanzo beans

- Pinch of salt and pepper

- 1 ½ C. orzo

- 4 C. water

Method:

- Fill a pot with water. Heat to boiling.

- Add orzo and cover. Cook 7 minutes until al dente.

- Drain water and pour orzo into a serving dish. Toss and set aside to cool.

- Toss herbs and onions in orzo, along with garbanzo beans and tomatoes.

- Add red wine vinaigrette tbsp by tbsp, seasoning with pepper and salt to achieve desired taste.

- Serve at room temperature or chill for a bit before consuming.

Crispy Peanut Eggplant Pasta

Serves: four

Ingredients:

- Pinch of salt and pepper

- 2 tbsp. balsamic vinegar

- 1 tbsp. oregano

- 3 tbsp. extra virgin olive oil

- ¼ C. nutritional yeast

- ½ C. toasted/chopped peanuts

- ¼ C. whole-grain flour

- ½ pound of chopped spinach

- 4 peeled/chopped cloves garlic

- 3-4 diced tomatoes

- ½ diced yellow onion

- 1 sliced eggplant

- 8 ounces whole-grain pasta

Method:

- Cook pasta in boiling water until al dente. Drain, rinse and toss with extra virgin olive oil. Set to the side.

- Combine oregano, pepper, salt, and flour together.

- Toss slices of eggplant in flour mixture and ensure they are evenly coated.

- Heat oil in a skillet and add slices of eggplant.

- Cook on both sides till tender. Put on a plate and set to the side.

- In the same skillet, sauté garlic and onion till brown. Add tomato and cook covered 4-5 minutes till tomatoes begin to break down.

- Add spinach and pasta.

- Turn heat to low and pour in pepper, salt, oregano, yeast, oil, and vinegar. Heat till pasta is warmed through.

- Serve pasta topped with slices of eggplant and hazelnuts.

Super Star Lentil Taco Salad

Serves: two

Ingredients:

- 1 sliced avocado

- 1 tsp. avocado oil

- ½ C. cilantro

- 1 C. broccoli

- 1 C. sliced bell pepper

- 1 C. sliced mushrooms

- 1 sliced red onion

- Pinch of salt

- 2 tbsp. balsamic vinegar

- 1 tsp. chili powder

- ½ tsp. pepper

- ½ tsp. turmeric

- 1 C. chopped tomatoes

- 3 C. organic vegetable broth
- 1 ½ C. brown or green dried lentils

Method:

- Bring to a boil pepper, turmeric, tomatoes, ½ tsp salt, and broth. Cover and reduce to simmer. Cook 15 minutes until lentils are soft.

- While lentils cook, warm up oil and add chili powder and veggies. Sauté till browned. Add cilantro, salt, and vinegar. Stir and take off heat.

- Once lentils are cooked, stir in anymore vinegar and salt if you desire.

- Place a big spoonful of lentils on serving plate, top with veggies and sliced avocado. Drizzle with hot sauce if you so choose.

Soups, Stews, and Curries

Soups, stews and curries are a great way to condense a variety of key plant-based foods into one tasty meal! They are also easy to make in large batches, put into containers and freeze/refrigerate for future consumption.

Sweet Potato and Red Bean Curry

Serves: two

Ingredients:

- 2 peeled/diced sweet potatoes
- 1 can red kidney beans
- 1 can diced tomatoes
- 1 ¾ C. organic vegetable stock
- 1 tbsp. peeled/grated ginger
- 2 minced garlic cloves
- 1 chopped green pepper
- Pinch of salt and pepper
- ¼ tsp. cayenne
- 1 tsp. turmeric
- ¾ tsp. cumin
- 1 tsp. coriander
- 1 tbsp. organic curry powder

- 1 chopped yellow onion
- 1 tbsp. extra virgin olive oil
- 2 C. brown rice

Method:

- Start cooking brown rice in boiling water for 15-20 minutes.

- Warm up extra virgin olive oil in a skillet. Add in onion, sautéing 5 minutes till soft.

- Mix in cayenne, turmeric, cumin, coriander, and curry powder. Then pour in ginger, garlic, bell pepper, cooking 30 seconds.

- Pour in stock and tomatoes and heat mixture to boiling.

- Turn down warmth to low and pour in sweet potatoes and beans. Sprinkle with pepper and salt to season.

- Cover and simmer 20 minutes till veggies become tender.

- Serve over cooked brown rice.

Avocado Soup

Serves: two

Ingredients:

- ¼ tsp. cayenne pepper
- Pinch of salt

- 1 tsp. cumin
- 1/3 C. fresh cilantro
- ¼ C. chopped chives
- 3 tbsp. fresh lemon juice
- 3 C. organic vegetable broth
- 3 avocados

Method:

- In a blender, process all soup components till smooth in texture.
- Cover blender cup and chill 2 hours.
- Serve chilled! Super simple!

Cream of Cauliflower Soup

Serves: two

Ingredients:

- 1 C. organic almond milk
- 6 tbsp. whole-grain flour
- ½ tsp. tarragon
- ½ tsp. dried basil
- Pinch of pepper and salt
- ¼ C. minced parsley

- 5 C. organic vegetable broth
- 1 head cauliflower
- ¼ C. coconut oil
- 2 minced cloves garlic
- 2 carrots
- 2 chopped onions

Method:

- Melt coconut oil.

- Sauté garlic, celery, onions, and carrots together till tender in a frying pan with 1 tsp. Coconut oil.

- Pour tarragon, basil, pepper, salt, parsley, broth, and cauliflower into the pan.

- Cover and simmer 30 minutes till veggies are tender.

- Mix in flour and almond milk. Heat to boiling and stir 2 minutes till the mixture becomes thickened.

- Take off heat. Serve with a garnish of tarragon. Enjoy!

Jackfruit "Chicken" Noodle Soup with Lima Beans

Serves: two

Ingredients:

- 8 C. water

- 1 C. dry organic noodles

- 2 bouillon cubes

- 1 garlic clove

- 1 onion

- ¼ C. dry lima beans

- 1 celery stalk

- 1 carrot

- 1 can of organic jackfruit in brine

Method:

- To make "chicken," drain can of jackfruit and pour in 2 cups of boiling water and 1 bouillon cube. Let sit for 60 minutes.

- While jackfruit is sitting cook lima beans for 5 minutes in boiling water, take off heat and let sit with lid on for 60 minutes also.

- Cook organic noodles in boiling water until ready.

- Warm up oil in a skillet. Pour in jackfruit and fry till browned. Save the jackfruit broth. Shred jackfruit.

- Place bouillon cube and reserved jackfruit broth into shredded jackfruit. Put in skillet and allow to simmer till liquid cooks away.

- To make soup, mix together cooked noodles and lima beans with broth and cooked jackfruit.

Chunky Potato Split Pea Soup

Serves: two

Ingredients:

- 1 tbsp. rice bran oil
- 2-3 tbsp. nutritional yeast
- 1 tsp. paprika
- Pinch pepper and salt
- 1 tbsp. balsamic vinegar
- 4 C. water
- 1 C. split peas
- 2 chopped russet potatoes
- 2 bay leaves
- ½ C. spinach
- 2 chopped mushrooms
- 1 chopped celery stalk
- 1 chopped carrot
- 1 yellow onion

Optional:

- 2 pieces whole-grain crusty bread

Method:

- Sauté water and split peas with bay leaves and onion. Warm till it boils. Turn down warmth and put on the lid. Cook 20-30 minutes till soft.

- Cook potatoes and carrot in boiling water until soft, add celery.

- Fry mushrooms and spinach with rice bran oil.

- Season split peas with yeast, paprika, balsamic vinegar, pepper, and salt.

- Add vegetables

- Serve soup with whole-grain crusty bread if you wish.

Potato Lentil Turmeric Soup

Serves: two

Ingredients:

- 1 tsp. turmeric

- 1 tbsp. rice bran oil

- Pinch of salt and pepper

- 1 tbsp. brown mustard seeds

- 1 tbsp. cumin seeds

- 4 C. organic vegetable broth

- 1 C. dried red lentils

- 1" piece of ginger

- 2 chopped cloves garlic

- 1 yellow onion

- 2 C. Yukon gold potatoes

Method:

- In a Dutch oven, warm up oil. Pour in mustard and cumin seeds. Heat 1-2 minutes till seeds start to pop. Ensure that they do not burn.

- Add ginger, garlic, and onion. Cook covered 2-3 minutes till onion softens.

- Add in red lentils and potatoes. Stir and pour in broth, heat to simmering.

- Cook covered on low 15-20 minutes till lentils soften.

- Add turmeric, pepper, and salt.
  You can eat soup chunky or use an immersion blender to create a smooth soup.

Sesame Sweet Potato Curry with Basil Rice

Serves: two

Ingredients:

- ¼ C. chopped basil

- Pinch of salt and pepper

- 2 C. organic jasmine rice + 3 ½ C. water

- ¼ C. toasted sesame seeds

- ¼ C. tahini

- 1-2 tbsp. soy sauce

- 1 tbsp. fresh lime juice
- 1 tbsp. extra virgin olive oil
- 1 tbsp. agave
- 1 tbsp. rice vinegar
- ½ C. cilantro
- 1 can organic coconut milk
- 1 bunch chopped green onion
- 1 sliced red cabbage
- ½ C. chopped mushrooms
- 1 cubed sweet potato
- 1 chopped hot chili
- 1" peeled/chopped ginger
- 2 chopped cloves garlic
- 2 diced shallots

Method:

- Cook organic jasmine rice in boiling water. Turn down heat. Simmer 10-20 minutes till fluffy. Mix in pinch of salt and ¼ C. basil.

- While rice cooks, sauté chili, ginger, garlic, and onion with tbsp. of extra virgin olive oil. Cook till softened.

- Add in mushrooms and sweet potato. Cook 2-3 minutes till mushrooms shrink.

- Pour in green onions, cabbage, and coconut milk. Cook covered 3-4 minutes till cabbage becomes soft.

- Stir in remaining recipe components, combining and adjusting seasonings as needed.

- Serve over basil organic jasmine rice and sprinkle with toasted sesame seeds. Drizzle with a bit of tahini.

Cauliflower Sweet Potato Mushroom Curry

Serves: two

Ingredients:

- ¼ C. chopped cilantro

- 1 tsp. lemon juice

- 1 tbsp. avocado oil

- Pinch of salt and pepper

- 1 tsp. turmeric

- 1 can organic coconut milk

- 1 ½ C. diced tomatoes

- 2 C. cauliflower florets

- 3-4 sliced mushrooms

- 2 C. diced sweet potato

- 1 chopped yellow onion
- 1 Serrano chili pepper
- 1 tbsp. chopped ginger
- 1 tbsp. pumpkin seeds
- 1 tbsp. cumin seeds
- 1 ½ C. brown rice

Method:

- In a deep skillet, mix 1 tbsp. avocado oil with pumpkin and cumin seeds. Heat till pumpkin seeds start to pop.

- Start cooking brown rice in boiling water for 15-20 minutes.

- Add onion, ginger, and chili. Sauté 2-3 minutes till onions are tender.

- Mix in mushrooms and sauté till soft.

- Add tomatoes. Cover and cook 3-4 minutes.

- Add turmeric, coconut milk, cauliflower, and sweet potato. Cover and cook 5-10 minutes till veggies become tender.

- Season with cilantro, lemon juice, pepper, and salt.

- Serve over cooked brown rice.

Perfect Potato and Pea Coconut Curry

Serves: two

Ingredients:

- 1 tbsp. rice bran oil
- ½ C. frozen peas
- ¼ C. chopped cilantro
- Pinch of agave
- 1 tsp. lemon juice
- Pinch of salt and pepper
- ½ tsp. turmeric
- 1 C. organic coconut milk
- 2-3 sliced mushrooms
- 1 diced russet potato
- 1 chopped clove garlic
- 1 diced yellow onion
- 1 deseeded chili pepper
- 1 tbsp. fresh ginger
- 1 tbsp. brown mustard seeds
- 1 tbsp. cumin seeds

Method:

- In a deep skillet, heat rice bran oil. Add cumin and mustard seeds. Cook 1-2 minutes till seeds begin to make a popping sound.

- Mix in ginger, onion, garlic, and pepper. Cook 2-3 minutes till softened.

- Add mushrooms and potato. Coat by stirring.

- Add pepper, turmeric, and coconut milk. Cover and cook 10-15 minutes till potatoes become soft.

- Add agave, salt, cilantro, peas, and lemon juice. Stir and cook 1-2 minutes.

- Serve and enjoy!

Tomato Potato Soup with Edamame

Serves: two

Ingredients:

- 1 chopped zucchini

- 1/3 C. chopped carrots

- 4 sliced mushrooms

- ½ C. edamame

- 2 stalks of chopped celery

- 1 tsp. thyme

- Pinch of salt and pepper

- 1 bay leaf

- 2 C. water

- 2 C. organic tomato soup

- 1/3 C. chopped onion
- 1-2 cloves of garlic

Method:

- Sauté onion with a bit of water till translucent. Stir in garlic.

- Add spices, bay leaf, water, and organic tomato soup. Pour in chopped zucchini, carrots, mushrooms, potato and celery. Cook on high till mixture starts to boil.

- Cover pot and turn down heat to let simmer. Let simmer 20 minutes till veggies start to become tender.

- Cook edamame in boiling water for 5 minutes, rinse and drain, start squeezing until edamame beans come out of shell.

- Pour half of soup mixture into a blender, and blend until creamy.

- Then add creamy soup back to soup pot. Mix with cooked edamame and serve!

Clean Eating Bowls

Clean eating bowls are extremely popular currently. They are fantastic if you don't necessarily enjoy cooking complicated meals, they are generally fairly simple and packed full of flavor and varying plant-based foods. You can mix and match your favorite items and work out your go to clean eating bowl for work lunches or on the weekend!

Simple Sushi Bowl

Serves: one

Ingredients:

- 1 tbsp. avocado oil

- 1 tbsp. organic rice vinegar

- Pinch of salt

- 3-4 tbsp. soy sauce

- ¼ C. sesame seeds

- 1 sliced sweet potato

- 1 chopped bunch kale

- ½ C. sliced mushrooms

- 1 ¾ C. water

- 1 C. brown sushi rice

Method:

- Cook rice in boiling water for 15-20 minutes.

- As rice cooks, sauté mushrooms with ½ tbsp. avocado oil. Once they have released the majority of fluids, add soy sauce and vinegar. Sprinkle with a pinch of salt and cook 2-3 minutes till crispy. Set aside on a plate.

- In the same pan, add ½ tbsp. of avocado oil and place sweet potato slices in an even layer. Allow to cook, soften, and brown. Then flip over. Sprinkle with salt as they cook. Take out of the pan and put to the side.

- Mix in soy sauce and greens to pan. Cook 1-2 minutes. Take out of the pan and put to the side.

- Toast sesame seeds in skillet till fragrant.

- Serve veggies over brown sushi rice and drizzle with soy sauce.

Garlic Baby Potato Bowl

Serves: one

Ingredients:

- 1/2 – ¾ C. water

- 1 tbsp. rosemary

- ½ tsp. thyme

- 1 tbsp. soy sauce

- Pinch of salt and pepper

- 2 tbsp. whole-grain flour

- 4 chopped mushrooms

- 3 tbsp. avocado oil

- 1 tsp. balsamic vinegar

- ¾ C. frozen peas

- 3 sliced sweet peppers

- 3 slices shallots

- 2 sliced summer squash

- 3 chopped cloves garlic

- ½ C. baby potatoes

Method:

- Wash potatoes. Place in a pot and pour enough water to cover potatoes. Heat pot till it begins to boil. Put on lid. Cook 10-20 minutes till tenderized.

- Pour out water, return potatoes to pot and toss with pepper, salt, garlic, and avocado oil.

- While potatoes cook, sauté veggies. Add peas and season with vinegar.

- For gravy, heat 2 tbsp of avocado oil and add mushrooms. Cook 3-4 minutes till browned. Then add flour and combine, cooking for 60 seconds. Add in salt and water. Stir and let cook till bubbly and thick.

- To serve, top potatoes with veggies and mushroom gravy. Enjoy!

Honeydew and Blackberry Bowl

Serves: one

Ingredients:

- ¼ C. chopped basil

- 1 tbsp. evaporated cane juice

- Pinch of salt and pepper

- 1 tsp. grated lime zest

- 2 tbsp. fresh lime juice

- 1 C. blackberries

- 1 C. cut up honeydew melon

Method:

- Add melon and ½ of blackberries to a serving bowl. Put in fridge to chill.

- In a pan on low warmth, add lime juice and zest, cane juice and 2 tbsp of water. Stir and cook till cane juice dissolves. Allow to cool to room temp.

- Combine remaining blackberries with lime juice mixture, pepper, salt, and 2 tbsp. of basil. Mash berries till sauce forms.

- Drizzle blackberry basil sauce over fruit. Garnish with basil if desired.

Curried Coconut Quinoa and Greens Bowl

Serves: two-four (depending on bowl sizes)

Ingredients:

Roasted Cauliflower:

- ¼ tsp. cayenne pepper
- 2 tbsp. melted coconut oil
- Pinch of salt
- 1 head cauliflower

Curried Coconut Quinoa with Greens:

- 4 C. baby arugula
- 1 tbsp. organic apple cider vinegar (with the 'mother')
- Pinch of salt
- 1/3 C. raisins
- 1 C. quinoa
- ½ C. water
- 1 can organic coconut milk
- ½ tsp. cardamom
- ½ tsp. curry powder

- 1 tsp. turmeric

- 1 tsp. ginger

- 1 chopped yellow onion

- 2 tsp. melted coconut oil

Method:

- Ensure oven is preheated to 425 degrees.

- Toss cauliflower florets with salt, cayenne, and coconut oil.

- Roast 25-30 minutes till edges are golden.

- Rise quinoa as it has a bit of a bitter flavor, cook quinoa in boiling water for 15-20 minutes. Then add in onion, cardamom, curry powder, ginger, and turmeric. Cook till fragrant.

- Bring mixture to boiling and add raisins, water, and coconut milk. Turn down heat and cook for 15 minutes.

- Mix up quinoa with a fork to fluff. Stir in greens, vinegar, and salt.

- Divide quinoa into bowls and top with roasted cauliflower.

Cauliflower Rice Bowl

Serves: two

Ingredients:

- ¼ tsp. garlic powder
- ¼ tsp. cayenne pepper
- 1 avocado
- Pinch of salt and pepper
- ¾ C. chickpeas
- 1 tsp. extra virgin olive oil
- 1 ½ C. cauliflower

Method:

- Ensure oven is preheated to 400 degrees.
- In a food processor, blend cauliflower until a rice forms.
- Warm up oil in a pan and place cauliflower into it. Mix up spices and then sprinkle over cauliflower. Cook 3-4 minutes.
- Add chickpeas and cook 5-7 minutes.
  Cut avocado in half. Lightly salt with pepper and salt.
- Once rice is heated through, scoop out and put into each avocado half.
- Bake 7-9 minutes.

- Remove and top with salsa, hot sauce, or other preferred toppings if you wish.

Dinner

Eggplant Parmesan

Serves: two

Ingredients:

Marinara Sauce:

- 1 can organic diced tomatoes
- ½ C. chopped fresh basil
- 1 tbsp. extra virgin olive oil
- Pinch of salt

Eggplant Parmesan:

- 1 tsp. organic cornstarch
- ½ C. organic unsweetened plain almond milk
- Pinch of salt
- 1 tsp. dried oregano
- 2 tbsp. vegan parmesan + more for serving
- 1 C. whole-grain bread crumbs
- ¼ C. whole-grain flour
- 1 eggplant

Method:

- Cut eggplant into thin oval pieces and sprinkle with salt. Place in a colander in a circular pattern to draw out the bitterness. Let sit 15 minutes then rinse and place on a towel. Place another towel on top and place a baking tray on top and put something heavy on the tray. Let dry 10 minutes.

- Ensure oven is preheated to 400 degrees. With foil, line a tray and grease with oil.

- Heat up a pot of water to boiling.

- Pour almond milk and cornstarch in a bowl. Mix.

- Place whole-grain flour in another bowl.

- Put oregano, parmesan, salt, and whole-grain breadcrumbs mixed together in another bowl.

- Once dry, dip eggplant in whole-grain flour, then almond milk, then breadcrumbs.

- Put onto the sheet. Bake 20-30 minutes.

- While eggplant bakes, prepare marinara in frying pan, add 1 tbsp. extra virgin olive oil, can of organic diced tomatoes and chopped basil with a pinch of salt.

- Pour marinara sauce over baked eggplant

- Serve with additional vegan parmesan if desired.

Hearty Lentil Bolognese

Serves: four

Ingredients:

- ¼ C. nutritional yeast
- ½ C. chopped basil
- ½ C. chopped parsley
- Pinch of salt and pepper
- 1 tbsp. agave
- ¾ C. dried brown or green lentils
- ½ C. chopped walnuts
- 1 tsp. thyme
- 1 tbsp. oregano
- 2 C. water
- 1 6-ounce organic can tomato paste
- 3 C. diced tomatoes
- ½ C. organic white or red wine
- 1 C. chopped mushrooms
- ½ C. diced celery
- 1 tbsp. extra virgin olive oil
- ½ C. diced carrot

- 3 chopped cloves garlic

- 1 diced yellow onion

- 8 ounces whole-grain pasta

Method:

- Cook pasta in boiling water until al dente.

- Warm up olive oil and sauté mushrooms in skillet, celery, carrots, garlic, and onion for 3-4 minutes.

- Once slightly soft, pour in wine and combine. Add tomatoes and cover. Cook 5-6 minutes till tomatoes begin to break down.

- Pour in organic tomato paste, water, oregano, thyme, and lentils and warm till it boils. Turn down warmth. Put on lid. Simmer 20 minutes till lentils soften, and sauce starts to thicken.

- Pour in agave, pepper, salt, parsley, basil, and yeast. Add walnuts close to the end of cooking.

- Once walnuts are added, turn off heat and stir to combine.

- Serve over pasta and with veggies.

Pumpkin Chipotle Chili with Sweet Potato Tortillas

Serves: four

Ingredients:

- 1 C. cooked black beans
- 2 tbsp. organic tomato paste
- 1 can organic pumpkin puree
- 3 C. water
- ½ C. quinoa
- 2 tbsp. diced/deseeded chipotle peppers
- ¼ tsp. cumin
- 1 tsp. ancho chili powder
- 2 tsp. soy sauce
- 1 diced carrot
- 1 diced bell pepper
- 2 minced cloves garlic
- ½ diced red onion
- 1 sliced avocado
- 4 sliced sweet potatoes
- 1 tbsp. rice bran oil

Method:

- Sauté onion in 1-2 tbsp of water. When soft, add in garlic and cook till a bit browned.

- Add in soy sauce, carrot, and bell pepper. Combine and then add chipotle pepper. Quickly combine. Add water if mixture starts to thicken too much.

- Add organic tomato paste, pumpkin, water, quinoa, and spices. Stir until well combined and turn up warmth to high.

- Once boiling, turn warmth to low. Simmer 20 minutes.

- Slice up your sweet potatoes into thin long strips and grill (if you have a grill) or fry with 1 tbsp. rice bran oil until golden brown, flipping every few minutes.

- When quinoa is cooked, pour in black beans and cook 5 more minutes.
  Serve alongside avocado and use your sliced grilled/fried sweet potato strips as tortilla chip substitutes. Devour!

Portobello Pot Roast

Serves: four

Ingredients:

- 1 sprig rosemary

- 4 sprigs thyme

- 2 tsp. organic vegan Worcestershire sauce

- Pinch of salt and pepper

- 4 carrots

- 4 potatoes

- 3 C. organic vegetable broth

- 1 tsp. basil

- 1 tsp. sage

- 3 tbsp. whole-grain flour

- 2 cloves garlic

- 1 sliced onion

- 4 sliced mushrooms

- ½ C. organic white wine

Method:

- Ensure oven is preheated to 350 degrees.

- Heat up ¼ cup of wine and place portobello mushroom slices into pan. Cook until browned. Make sure to continuously move them around to prevent burning.

- Pour in remaining wine and then add garlic and onion. Caramelize till brown.

- Remove onions and set to side.

- Mix basil, sage, and flour together. Then stir in ¼ cup of broth till paste is formed. Pour into pan. Stir till gravy is created.

- Once boiling, turn off heat and add in seasonings.

- Place pepper, salt, carrots, potatoes, and the vegan organic Worcestershire sauce into gravy. If you need to add more broth, feel free to do so.

- Add sliced onions and mushroom to gravy.

- Ladle into a casserole dish, layering sprigs of thyme and rosemary.

- Put lid on and bake 1 hour.

Mashed Cauliflower and Green Bean Casserole

Serves: two

Ingredients:

- 1 diced onion

- 2 C. of trimmed green beans

- Pinch of salt and pepper

- 1 head of cauliflower

- ½ C. nutritional yeast

- ¾ C. organic coconut milk

- 1 tbsp. extra virgin olive oil

Method:

- Ensure oven is preheated to 400 degrees.

- Cut cauliflower into florets.

- Steam within a microwave for 8 minutes.

- Warm extra virgin olive oil in a pan. Add green beans and onions to pan and cook.

- Once cauliflower is steamed, pour into a blender with pepper, salt, yeast, and coconut milk. Blend till smooth.

- In a casserole dish, layer green bean mix with mashed cauliflower.

- Bake 15 minutes. Enjoy!

Zucchini Noodles with Portobello Bolognese

Serves: four

Ingredients:

- 4 zucchinis

- ½ C. basil leaves

- ¼ tsp. red pepper

- 2 tsp. oregano

- 1 tbsp. organic tomato paste

- Pepper and salt

- 3 minced cloves garlic

- ½ C. minced yellow onion

- ½ C. minced celery

- ½ C. minced carrot

- 6 portobello mushrooms

- 3 tbsp. extra virgin olive oil

- 1 can organic diced tomatoes

Method:

- Wash mushrooms caps well. Remove stems and scrape off gills. Finely chop.

- Warm up 2 tbsp extra virgin olive oil. Sauté garlic, onion, celery, carrots, and mushrooms together. Season with pepper and salt. Cook 8-10 minutes till veggies become tender.

- Mix in organic tomato paste and cook 2 minutes.

- Mix in red pepper, basil, oregano, and organic diced tomatoes. Simmer 15 minutes till a thick sauce forms.

- Season more if you desire.

- While sauce cooks, spiralize zucchini into noodles with a spiralizer.

- In another pan, heat up remaining extra virgin olive oil. Cook noodles 2 minutes. Season with pepper and salt.

- Divide zucchini noodles among serving bowls and ladle sauce over top.

Pumpkin Cannelloni with Cashew Cream

Serves: two

Ingredients:

Cashew Cream:

- 1-2 tsp. red pepper flakes
- 2 C. organic tomato sauce
- 6 organic green lentil lasagne sheets
- Pinch of salt
- 2 tsp. nutritional yeast
- 1 garlic clove
- 1 C. boiling water
- ½ C. raw cashews

Filling:

- 1/8 tsp. pepper
- Pinch of salt
- 1 tsp. garlic powder
- 1 tsp. onion powder
- 1 tsp. nutritional yeast
- 1 can organic pumpkin puree

Method:

- To make cashew cream, soak cashews in boiling water for half an hour. Drain water but reserve ½ cup of water.

- In a blender, mix reserved water with salt, yeast, garlic, and cashews till creamy. Place in fridge till ready to use.

- Bring a pot of water to boiling, add salt. Place lasagne sheets in pot and cook 10 minutes.

- Make filling as pasta cooks. Mix all filling components together.

- Once pasta is cooked, drain and run under cold water.

- Ensure oven is preheated to 375 degrees.

- Mix red pepper flakes with tomato sauce and pour into bottom of baking dish.

- Then pour half of cashew cream over sauce.

- Put about a tbsp of filling into each pasta sheet and roll. Arrange pasta rolls in dish and cover with more tomato sauce and cashew cream.
  Cover with foil and bake 45 minutes.

- Drizzle with more cashew cream when serving.

Side Dishes and Snacks

Zucchini and Corn Fritters

Serves: two

Ingredients:

- 1 tsp. thyme
- 2 tsp. cumin
- Pinch of salt and pepper
- 1 ¼ C. organic chickpea flour
- 3 minced garlic cloves
- ¾ C. chopped green onions
- 1 ½ C. corn kernels
- 1 tbsp. rice bran oil
- 1 tsp. avocado oil
- 4 C. shredded zucchini
- 1 sliced avocado
- ½ C. black beans

Method:

- Mix together pepper, salt, thyme, oregano, cumin, chickpea flour, green onions, corn, and zucchini. Let sit 5 minutes to absorb moisture from zucchini.

- Warm up a skillet and grease with rice bran oil.

- Spoon ¼ cup of zucchini mixture into skillet, cooking 3-5 minutes on each side until golden brown.

- Rinse black beans and heat up in a frying pan with 1 tsp. avocado oil for 60 seconds.

- Serve alongside sliced avocado and black beans!

Cauliflower Mac n' Cheese

Serves: two

Ingredients:

- ½ tsp. garlic powder

- ½ tsp. onion powder

- 1 tbsp. lemon juice

- Pinch of salt and pepper

- 1/3 C. water

- 1/3 C. extra virgin olive oil

- ½ C. nutritional yeast

- 2 peeled/chopped carrots

- 1 head cauliflower

- 4 C. whole-grain macaroni

Optional:

- Sprinkle of parmesan cheese

- Sprinkle of paprika

Method:

- Cook whole-grain macaroni in boiling water, drain and set to the side.

- Heat pot of water to boiling. Place cauliflower and carrots in the pot. Cook 10-15 minutes till soft. Pour out water and then place in a blender.

- Pour in pepper, salt, garlic powder, onion powder, yeast, lemon juice, water, and oil in with veggies in a blender. Blend until smooth.

- Pour cauliflower cheese sauce over pasta. Mix.

- Serve with a liberal sprinkling of vegan parmesan and paprika if you wish.

Mediterranean Pasta Salad

Serves: four

Ingredients:

- ¾ C. minced parsley

- 4 diced scallions

- ¾ C. diced olives

- ½ yellow bell pepper, sliced

- ½ red bell pepper, sliced

- 1 C. chopped cucumber

- 8 ounces whole-grain pasta

Dressing:

- 2 minced cloves garlic

- Pinch of salt and pepper

- 2 tsp. agave

- 2 tbsp. tahini

- ¼ C. organic red wine vinegar

- ½ C. extra virgin olive oil

Method:

- Cook whole-grain pasta in boiling water. Drain and under cold water, rinse. Toss noodles with a bit of olive oil so that noodles do not stick together.

- Place parsley, scallions, olives, bell peppers, cucumbers, and red onions in a bowl. Pour pasta in a bowl and toss all ingredients together.

- Mix up dressing components in a separate bowl until creamy.

- Pour half of dressing over pasta mixture, tossing well. Add more dressing if needed. Enjoy!

Oven-baked Sesame Fries

Serves: two

Ingredients:

- 1 tbsp. nutritional yeast

- 1 tbsp. organic potato starch
- Pinch of salt and pepper
- 2 tbsp. sesame seeds
- 2 tbsp. avocado oil
- 2 cups diced Yukon potatoes

Method:

- Ensure oven is preheated to 425 degrees.
- Oil a baking tray.
- Cut up potatoes into wedges.
- Mix all components together minus the potatoes.
- Place potatoes on baking tray and toss with other component mixture. Drizzle with more oil if needed.
- Bake potatoes 20-25 minutes, making sure to flip halfway through.
- When golden and crispy you are ready to serve!

Buffalo Cauliflower Wings and Dip

Serves: two

Ingredients:

- ¼ C. raw cashews
- ¼ tsp. dill
- 1 tsp. parsley
- 1 tsp. organic apple cider vinegar (with the 'mother')
- Pinch of salt and pepper
- ¼ tsp. onion powder
- ¼ tsp. garlic powder
- 1/8 C. organic almond milk
- ½ C. vegan mayonnaise
- ½ C. hot sauce
- 1 tsp. vegan butter
- Pinch of salt
- ½ tsp. onion powder
- 1 tsp. garlic powder
- ½ C. water
- ½ C. + 2 tbsp. whole-grain flour

- 1 head cauliflower

Method:

- Ensure oven is preheated to 450 degrees.

- Chop cauliflower into wing sized bites.

- Mix salt, garlic and onion powders, water, and flour together.

- Toss cauliflower pieces with flour mixture.

- Put cauliflower on a tray lined with parchment paper. Cook 8 minutes.

- While cauliflower cooks, make the hot sauce by mixing vegan butter and hot sauce together.

- Take out cauliflower. Toss in hot sauce mixture and pop back in the oven to cook 8 more minutes.

- Take cauliflower out of the oven. Toss cauliflower once more in hot sauce mixture.

- Cook 25-30 more minutes till crisp.

- To make the dip, combine herbs, vinegar, garlic and onion powders, almond milk, and vegan mayonnaise in a blender on high speed. Add cashews and blend slightly.

- Adjust taste with pepper and salt if needed. Chill mixture till wings are ready.

- Take out cauliflower. Let cool 5 minutes before consuming. Serve with dip!

Sunflower Chive "Cheese" Cucumbers

Serves: two

Ingredients:

- ½ C. water
- 2 tbsp. lemon juice
- 2 tbsp. nutritional yeast
- 1 chopped garlic clover
- 1 chopped handful chives
- 2 tbsp. chopped red onion
- Pinch of salt
- 1 C. raw sunflower seeds
- 4 cucumbers

Method:

- In a food processor, add salt and sunflower seeds. Process until a fine powder forms.
- Add remaining recipe components minus cucumbers. Process 1-2 minutes till creamy.
- Peel cucumber, alternating rows to create a striped effect. Slice into 1-1/2" pieces.
- Spread spoonful of "cheese" on each cucumber.
- Sprinkle with chives. Serve!

Cheesy Roasted Tahini Brussels Sprouts

Serves: two

Ingredients:

- ½ tsp. garlic powder
- Pinch of salt
- ½ tsp. paprika
- 2 tsp. lemon juice
- 1 tbsp. nutritional yeast
- 1 tbsp. extra virgin olive oil
- 1 tbsp. warm water
- 1 tbsp. tahini
- 2 C. raw brussels sprouts

Method:

- Ensure oven is preheated to 400 degrees. With parchment paper, line a baking sheet.
- Combine yeast, oil, garlic powder, lemon juice, paprika, salt, water, and tahini till smooth.
- Toss Brussels sprouts with sauce till coated evenly.
- Lay the sprouts on the sheet.
  Top with additional salt, pepper, and yeast.
- Bake 30-35 minutes. Turn halfway through roasting.

- Remove from oven when lightly browned. Enjoy!

Roasted Spring Veggie Plate

Serves: two

Ingredients:

- Pinch of herbs you desire: Oregano, thyme, rosemary, etc.

- Liberal amount of pepper and salt

- 1 tbsp. avocado oil

- Spring veggies you desire: zucchini, leeks, broccoli, green onion, asparagus, etc.

Method:

- Ensure oven is preheated to 425 degrees.

- Drizzle baking sheet with avocado oil.

- Place veggies in an even layer on baking tray. Dash veggies with pepper, salt, and herbs of choice. Toss to coat everything well.

- Bake 10 minutes. Veggies should be bright in color and tender.

- Season to taste before serving.

Smoky Roasted Red Pepper Hummus

Serves: two

Ingredients:

- ¼ tsp. chili powder

- ¼ tsp. cumin

- Pinch of salt and pepper

- 1 tbsp. tahini

- ¼ C. roasted red peppers + ½ tsp. juice from jar

- 1 C. cooked chickpeas

- ¼ C. dried parsley flakes

- 1 tbsp. chopped chives

- Dash of garlic powder

Methods:

- In a blender, add all components except parsley and chives. Process well.

- Adjust seasonings if you desire.

- Chill for 20 minutes.

- Pour into a bowl and garnish with parsley and chives.

Jalapeno Corn Bread

Serves: two

Ingredients:

- 1 can organic sweet corn

- 1 diced jalapeno

- 1 tsp. baking powder

- 1 tsp. baking soda

- ½ tsp. salt

- 1 C. organic ground cornmeal

- 1 C. whole-grain flour

- ¼ tsp. stevia or 2 tbsp. brown sugar

- 2 tbsp. rice bran oil

- 2 pureed cored apples (acting applesauce)

- 1 ½ tbsp. organic apple cider vinegar (with the 'mother')

- 1 C. organic almond milk

Method:

- Ensure oven is preheated to 400 degrees.

- Mix apple cider vinegar with almond milk. Put to the side to sit.

- Put cored apples into a food processor and blend.

- Mix stevia/brown sugar, rice bran oil, and apple-sauce together.

- Mix all dry recipe components together.

- Pour vinegar milk into applesauce mixture and stir. Then incorporate dry mixture.

- Pour mixture into a dish. Bake 30 minutes.

Desserts and Treats

We can't enjoy desserts and treats on a plant-based diet, right? Wrong! The below recipes are healthy and delicious. Stevia, as you have probably seen pop-up throughout the previous recipes is a natural plant based sweetener extracted from the leaves of the plant species Selvia Rebaudiana. If you do not have this ingredient, brown sugar or coconut sugar can also substitute. Of course everything in moderation is key.

Date and Coconut Balls

Serves: four

Ingredients:

- 1 tbsp. chia seeds

- 1/3 C. cacao powder

- 1/3 C. coconut oil

- ½ C. + 1/3 C. shredded coconut

- 1 C. ground almond flour

- 12 Medjool dates

Method:

- Soak dates in a bowl of water for 1 hour. Drain and remove pips.

- In a blender, blend together chia seeds, cacao powder, coconut oil, ½ cup shredded coconut, ground almond poweder, and dates.

- Pour mixture into a bowl and let chia seeds become soft.

- Pour remaining 1/3 cup shredded coconut into a shallow dish.

- Roll mixture into tbsp sized balls and roll into coconut.

- Chill 1 hour and enjoy!

Vegan Banana Bread

Serves: two

Ingredients:

- ½ C. melted coconut oil

- 2 tbsp. ground flaxseeds

- 1 tsp. baking soda

- 1/3 C. organic unsweetened almond milk

- 1 tsp. vanilla extract

- 1 1/3 C. mashed ripe bananas

- Pinch of salt

- 1 tsp. stevia or ¾ C. brown sugar

- 2 C. whole-grain flour

Method:

- Ensure oven is preheated to 350 degrees. Grease loaf pan with coconut oil.

- Add flaxseed to 1/3 cup of water. Let stand till thick. Combine.

- Whisk salt, baking soda, stevia/brown sugar, and flour together. Then mix in vanilla, banana, flaxseed mixture, almond milk, and coconut oil.

- In a the greased loaf pan, pour in batter.

- Bake 60-65 minutes.

Frozen Blueberry Coconut Yogurt

Serves: four

Ingredients:

- 1 1/3 C. ripe bananas

- 1 tsp. vanilla extract

- 1/3 C. organic almond milk

- Pinch of salt

- 1 tsp. baking soda

- 1 tsp. stevia or ¾ C. brown sugar

- 2 tbsp. ground flaxseed

- ½ C. melted coconut oil

- 2 C. whole-grain flour

Method:

- Ensure oven is preheated to 350 degrees. Flour and oil a 9x5" loaf pan.

- Sprinkle flaxseed into a 1/3 cup of water and let stand 5 minutes. Stir.

- Mix salt, baking soda, stevia/brown sugar, and flour together. Then mix in vanilla, bananas, flaxseed mixture, almond milk, and oil till combined.

- Into a greased loaf pan, pour batter.
  Bake 60-65 minutes.

- Set aside to cool off for 15 minutes before attempting to cut and devour!

Muesli Almond Bar

Serves: four

Ingredients:

- 1 C. dates

- ¾ C. slivered almonds

- 2 tsp. vanilla extract

- 2 tsp. stevia or 2 C. brown sugar

- ¾ C. coconut oil

- ½ tsp. cinnamon

- Pinch of salt

- 1 ½ tsp. baking powder

- ¾ C. whole-grain flour

- 2 ¾ C. whole-grain muesli

Method:

- Ensure oven is preheated to 350 degrees.

- Grind up 1 ¼ cups of whole-grain muesli in a food processor.

- Mix muesli, flour, cinnamon, salt, and baking powder.

- In another bowl, beat coconut oil and stevia/brown sugar together with electric mixer till fluffy. Mix in vanilla extract. Then mix in muesli mixture. Fold in dates and almonds.

- Spread batter evenly into greased dish and top with additional muesli.

- Bake 35 minutes, ensuring to turn halfway through.

- Allow to cool and cut bars. Enjoy!

Sweet Potato Brownies

Serves: four

Ingredients:

- ½ C. creamy peanut butter

- 1/3 C. dark non-dairy chocolate chips

- ½ C. organic maple syrup

- ½ C. organic oat flour

- ½ C. ground almond flour

- 10 tbsp. cocoa powder

- 2 cups cut up sweet potatoes

Method:

- Roast potatoes till soft.

- Ensure oven is preheated to 350 degrees.

- In a food processor, process cooked potatoes till smooth.
  Pour in syrup, organic oat flour, and ground almond flour. Process till smooth.

- Pour in almond milk a tbsp at a time. Then add chocolate chips. Process for a few seconds to combine.

- Pour brown mixture into pan.
  Bake 25-30 minutes.

- Take out of the oven and spread peanut butter over the top while warm.

- Put in fridge to cool.

Zucchini and Carrot Muffins

Serves: four

Ingredients:

- ½ - ¾ C. raisins
- ½ tsp. nutmeg
- 2 tsp. cinnamon
- 3 C. whole-grain flour
- Pinch of salt
- 2 tsp. baking soda
- 2 tsp. vanilla extract
- ¾ C. aquafaba (aka chickpea water - egg replacement)
- 1 tsp. stevia or 1C. brown sugar
- 2 pureed cored apples (acting applesauce)
- 1/3 C. melted vegan butter
- 1 C. grated carrots
- 2 C. grated zucchini

Method:

- Ensure oven is preheated to 350 degrees. Line muffin tray with liners.

- Use an electric hand mixer to whip the aquafaba to desired thickness and then add stevia/brown sugar and vanilla extract.

- Add grated zucchini and carrots to stevia/brown sugar, aquafaba, and vanilla mixture.

- Mix remaining dry components and spices together, then add them to egg mixture. Combine well.

- Fold in raisins.

- Use an ice cream scoop to spoon batter into liners. Fill to the top.

- Bake 18-20 minutes.

- Put cored apples into a food processor and blend.

- Top with applesauce!

Chocolate Chip Banana Bites

Ingredients:

- ¼ C. dark non-dairy chocolate chips

- ¼ C. rolled oats

- ½ ripe banana

- 2 tbsp. melted coconut oil

- 2 tbsp. agave

- 1 tsp. vanilla extract

- 1 tbsp. ground flaxseed

- ¼ tsp. cinnamon

- Pinch of salt

- ¾ C. organic rolled oats

Method:

- Blend ¾ cup rolled oats in a food processor.

- Pour in remaining recipe components into the processor, minus chips and remaining oats.

- Add chips and remaining oats. Stir well.

- Form mixture into balls. Place in fridge to set.

Chocolate Avocado Pudding

Serves: two

Ingredients:

- 1 ½ tbsp. coconut shreds

- 1 tbsp. agave

- 1 tbsp. coconut sugar

- 2 ½ tbsp. cocoa powder

- ½ tsp. salt

- 2 ripe bananas

Method:

- In a food processor, pour in all recipe components. Blend until smooth.

- Sprinkle with shredded coconut to serve. Super Easy!

No Bake Peanut Butter Cups

Serves: four

Ingredients:

- 1 tbsp. ground flaxseed

- 2 tbsp. organic maple syrup

- 1 C. peanut butter

- 1 ½ C. organic rolled oats

- ½ C. dried cranberries

- ½ C. dark non-dairy chocolate chips

Method:

- In a bowl, combine all recipe components minus chocolate chips.
  Melt chocolate chips and mix half of them into the mixture.
- Roll dough into balls.

- Lightly grease a muffin tin. Push balls into each section.

- Coat the cups with remaining chocolate.
  Chill for 1 hour.

Peanut Butter Sandwich Cookies

Serves: two

Ingredients:

- 1 C. whole-grain flour

- 3 tbsp. organic rolled oats

- ½ tsp. cinnamon

- ½ tsp. baking soda

- Pinch of salt

- ¼ C. water

- 2 tbsp. flaxseeds

- 2 ½ tbsp. vanilla extract

- ½ tsp. stevia or 1/2 C. brown sugar

- 1/3 C. creamy peanut butter + ½ C. for filling

- ½ C. coconut oil

Method:

- Ensure oven is preheated to 350 degrees. With parchment paper, line a baking sheet.

- Combine stevia/brown sugar, 1/3 cup peanut butter, and coconut oil together, creaming with a fork.

- Pour water, flaxseeds, and vanilla to mixture. Mix well.

- Add flour, oats, cinnamon, and baking soda. Combine.

- Roll mixture into balls. Put balls on sheet. Flatten with hand.

- Bake 12-15 minutes till lightly browned and crisp.

- Once cooled, coat bottom of one cookie with peanut butter. Attach to another cookie to make a sandwich.

Persimmon Bread

Serves: two

Ingredients:

- 2 tsp. cinnamon
- ½ tsp. clove
- ½ tsp. nutmeg
- Pinch of salt
- 1 tsp. baking soda
- ½ tsp. baking powder
- 1 ¾ C. whole-grain flour
- 1 C. persimmon puree
- 2 pureed cored apples (acting applesauce)
- 1 tsp. stevia or ¾ C. brown sugar
- ¾ C. rice bran oil

Method:

- Ensure oven is preheated to 350 degrees. Prepare a loaf pan by greasing sides with rice bran oil.

- Place the cored apples in a food pressor and blend.

- Blend oil and stevia/brown sugar together. Then add applesauce and persimmon puree. Combine.

- Add in spices, baking soda, and powder. Incorporate well.

- Pour mixture into loaf pan.

- Bake 1 hour. Enjoy!

4-Ingredient Chocolate Pie

Ingredients:

- 1 vegan graham cracker crust

- 2 tsp. vanilla extract

- 1 packed organic silken tofu

- 12 ounce bag of dark non-dairy semisweet chocolate chips

Method:

- Melt chocolate chips in microwave 45-60 seconds till smooth.

- In a blender, blend tofu till creamy. Pour in vanilla and melted chocolate. Blend well.

- Add tofu chocolate mixture to pie crust.

Place in freezer for 90 minutes. Enjoy!

Conclusion

Thank you for reading my book *Plant-Based Diet Cookbook* and congratulations for making it through to the end.

I hope that the contents of this book were able to demonstrate to you that getting back to the basics of eating is highly realistic! I hope that I was able to answer many of your inquiries in regards to a plant-based diet, as well as find the tools you need to reach your goal of incorporating more goodness in your diet and exterminating the things that only inhibit you from feeling your absolute best.

The next step is to put the knowledge you have absorbed from this cookbook into play. Did some recipes catch your eye? Make and try those out first! You will find as you make your way through the recipes within this book that it will become easier to implement delicious and healthy plant-based food items!

Why not fuel a beautiful mind, body and soul with a gorgeous array of consumable colors? It is time to make a positive lifestyle change and discover the rainbow of healthy whole foods.

If you found this book useful and helpful in any way, please take the time to leave a review on Amazon. It is much appreciated!